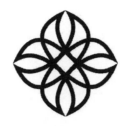

this

PLANNER

BELONGS TO:

_____

LIVE A HAPPY ORGANISED LIFE

2020

2019

JANUARY

S	M	T	W	T	F	S
		1	2	3	4	5
6	7	8	9	10	11	12
13	14	15	16	17	18	19
20	21	22	23	24	25	26
27	28	29	30	31		

FEBRUARY

S	M	T	W	T	F	S
					1	2
3	4	5	6	7	8	9
10	11	12	13	14	15	16
17	18	19	20	21	22	23
24	25	26	27	28		

MARCH

S	M	T	W	T	F	S
31					1	2
3	4	5	6	7	8	9
10	11	12	13	14	15	16
17	18	19	20	21	22	23
24	25	26	27	28	29	30

APRIL

S	M	T	W	T	F	S
	1	2	3	4	5	6
7	8	9	10	11	12	13
14	15	16	17	18	19	20
21	22	23	24	25	26	27
28	29	30				

MAY

S	M	T	W	T	F	S
			1	2	3	4
5	6	7	8	9	10	11
12	13	14	15	16	17	18
19	20	21	22	23	24	25
26	27	28	29	30	31	

JUNE

S	M	T	W	T	F	S
30						1
2	3	4	5	6	7	8
9	10	11	12	13	14	15
16	17	18	19	20	21	22
23	24	25	26	27	28	29

JULY

S	M	T	W	T	F	S
	1	2	3	4	5	6
7	8	9	10	11	12	13
14	15	16	17	18	19	20
21	22	23	24	25	26	27
28	29	30	31			

AUGUST

S	M	T	W	T	F	S
				1	2	3
4	5	6	7	8	9	10
11	12	13	14	15	16	17
18	19	20	21	22	23	24
25	26	27	28	29	30	31

SEPTEMBER

S	M	T	W	T	F	S
1	2	3	4	5	6	7
8	9	10	11	12	13	14
15	16	17	18	19	20	21
22	23	24	25	26	27	28
29	30					

OCTOBER

S	M	T	W	T	F	S
		1	2	3	4	5
6	7	8	9	10	11	12
13	14	15	16	17	18	19
20	21	22	23	24	25	26
27	28	29	30	31		

NOVEMBER

S	M	T	W	T	F	S
					1	2
3	4	5	6	7	8	9
10	11	12	13	14	15	16
17	18	19	20	21	22	23
24	25	26	27	28	29	30

DECEMBER

S	M	T	W	T	F	S
1	2	3	4	5	6	7
8	9	10	11	12	13	14
15	16	17	18	19	20	21
22	23	24	25	26	27	28
29	30	31				

2020

JANUARY

S	M	T	W	T	F	S
			1	2	3	4
5	6	7	8	9	10	11
12	13	14	15	16	17	18
19	20	21	22	23	24	25
26	27	28	29	30	31	

FEBRUARY

S	M	T	W	T	F	S
						1
2	3	4	5	6	7	8
9	10	11	12	13	14	15
16	17	18	19	20	21	22
23	24	25	26	27	28	29

MARCH

S	M	T	W	T	F	S
1	2	3	4	5	6	7
8	9	10	11	12	13	14
15	16	17	18	19	20	21
22	23	24	25	26	27	28
29	30	31				

APRIL

S	M	T	W	T	F	S
			1	2	3	4
5	6	7	8	9	10	11
12	13	14	15	16	17	18
19	20	21	22	23	24	25
26	27	28	29	30		

MAY

S	M	T	W	T	F	S
31					1	2
3	4	5	6	7	8	9
10	11	12	13	14	15	16
17	18	19	20	21	22	23
24	25	26	27	28	29	30

JUNE

S	M	T	W	T	F	S
	1	2	3	4	5	6
7	8	9	10	11	12	13
14	15	16	17	18	19	20
21	22	23	24	25	26	27
28	29	30				

JULY

S	M	T	W	T	F	S
			1	2	3	4
5	6	7	8	9	10	11
12	13	14	15	16	17	18
19	20	21	22	23	24	25
26	27	28	29	30	31	

AUGUST

S	M	T	W	T	F	S
30	31					1
2	3	4	5	6	7	8
9	10	11	12	13	14	15
16	17	18	19	20	21	22
23	24	25	26	27	28	29

SEPTEMBER

S	M	T	W	T	F	S
		1	2	3	4	5
6	7	8	9	10	11	12
13	14	15	16	17	18	19
20	21	22	23	24	25	26
27	28	29	30			

OCTOBER

S	M	T	W	T	F	S
				1	2	3
4	5	6	7	8	9	10
11	12	13	14	15	16	17
18	19	20	21	22	23	24
25	26	27	28	29	30	31

NOVEMBER

S	M	T	W	T	F	S
1	2	3	4	5	6	7
8	9	10	11	12	13	14
15	16	17	18	19	20	21
22	23	24	25	26	27	28
29	30					

DECEMBER

S	M	T	W	T	F	S
		1	2	3	4	5
6	7	8	9	10	11	12
13	14	15	16	17	18	19
20	21	22	23	24	25	26
27	28	29	30	31		

JANUARY 2020

SUNDAY	MONDAY	TUESDAY	WEDNESDAY
			1 NEW YEAR'S DAY
5	6	7	8
12	13	14	15
19	20 MARTIN LUTHER KING JR. DAY	21	22
26	27	28	29

Yoga is the perfect opportunity to be curious about who you are.

- Jason Crandell

THURSDAY	FRIDAY	SATURDAY	NOTES
2	3	4	
9	10	11	
16	17	18	
23	24	25	
30	31		

FEBRUARY 2020

SUNDAY	MONDAY	TUESDAY	WEDNESDAY
2 GROUNDHOG DAY	3	4	5
9	10	11	12
16	17 PRESIDENTS' DAY	18	19
23	24	25	26

Let your practice be a celebration of life.

- Seido Lee deBarros

THURSDAY	FRIDAY	SATURDAY	NOTES
		1	
6	7	8	
13	14 VALENTINE'S DAY	15	
20	21	22	
27	28	29	

MARCH 2020

SUNDAY	MONDAY	TUESDAY	WEDNESDAY
1	2	3	4
8	9	10	11
15	16	17 ST. PATRICK'S DAY	18
22	23	24	25
29	30	31	

In truth, yoga doesn't take time it gives time.

- Ganga White

THURSDAY	FRIDAY	SATURDAY	NOTES
5	6	7	
12	13	14	
19	20	21	
26	27	28	

APRIL 2020

SUNDAY	MONDAY	TUESDAY	WEDNESDAY
			1
5	6	7	8
12 EASTER DAY	13	14	15 TAX DAY
19	20	21	22
26	27	28	29

The longest journey of any person is the journey inward.

- Dag Hammarskjold

THURSDAY	FRIDAY	SATURDAY	NOTES
2	3	4	
9	10	11	
16	17	18	
23	24	25	
30			

MAY
2020

SUNDAY	MONDAY	TUESDAY	WEDNESDAY
31			
3	4	5 CINCO DE MAYO	6
10 MOTHER'S DAY	11	12	13
17	18	19	20
24	25 MEMORIAL DAY	26	27

The attitude of gratitude is the highest yoga.

- Yogi Bhajan

THURSDAY	FRIDAY	SATURDAY	NOTES
	1	2	
7	8	9	
14	15	16	
21	22	23	
28	29	30	

JUNE 2020

SUNDAY	MONDAY	TUESDAY	WEDNESDAY
	1	2	3
7	8	9	10
14	15	16	17
21 FATHER'S DAY	22	23	24
28	29	30	

Meditation is a way for nourishing and blossoming the divinity within you.

- Amit Ray

THURSDAY	FRIDAY	SATURDAY	NOTES
4	5	6	
11	12	13	
18	19	20	
25	26	27	

JULY 2020

SUNDAY	MONDAY	TUESDAY	WEDNESDAY
			1
5	6	7	8
12	13	14	15
19	20	21	22
26	27	28	29

The most important pieces of equipment you need for doing yoga are your body and your mind.

- Rodney Yee

THURSDAY	FRIDAY	SATURDAY	NOTES
2	3 INDEPENDENCE DAY (OBSERVED)	4 INDEPENDENCE DAY	_____
9	10	11	_____
16	17	18	_____
23	24	25	_____
30	31		_____

AUGUST 2020

SUNDAY	MONDAY	TUESDAY	WEDNESDAY
30	31		
2	3	4	5
9	10	11	12
16	17	18	19
23	24	25	26

Yoga is the journey of the self, through the self, to the self.

- The Bhagavad Gita

THURSDAY	FRIDAY	SATURDAY	NOTES
		1	_____
			_____
6	7	8	_____
			_____
13	14	15	_____
			_____
20	21	22	_____
			_____
27	28	29	_____

SEPTEMBER 2020

SUNDAY	MONDAY	TUESDAY	WEDNESDAY
		1	2
6	7 LABOR DAY	8	9
13	14	15	16
20	21	22	23
27	28	29	30

Nature does not hurry, yet everything is accomplished.

- Lao Tzu

THURSDAY	FRIDAY	SATURDAY	NOTES
3	4	5	
10	11	12	
17	18	19	
24	25	26	

OCTOBER 2020

SUNDAY	MONDAY	TUESDAY	WEDNESDAY
4	5	6	7
11	12 COLUMBUS DAY	13	14
18	19	20	21
25	26	27	28

The future depends on what we do in the present.

– Mahatma Gandhi

THURSDAY	FRIDAY	SATURDAY	NOTES
1	2	3	
8	9	10	
15	16	17	
22	23	24	
29	30	31 HALLOWEEN	

NOVEMBER 2020

SUNDAY	MONDAY	TUESDAY	WEDNESDAY
1	2	3 ELECTION DAY	4
8	9	10	11 VETERAN'S DAY
15	16	17	18
22	23	24	25
29	30		

Yoga does not transform the way we see things, it transforms the person who sees.

- B.K.S Iyengar

THURSDAY	FRIDAY	SATURDAY	NOTES
5	6	7	_____
			_____
			_____
12	13	14	_____
			_____
			_____
19	20	21	_____
			_____
			_____
26	27	28	_____
THANKSGIVING DAY	BLACK FRIDAY		_____
			_____

DECEMBER 2020

SUNDAY	MONDAY	TUESDAY	WEDNESDAY
		1	2
6	7	8	9
13	14	15	16
20	21	22	23
27	28	29	30

Remember to breathe. It is after all, the secret of life.

- Gregory Maguire

THURSDAY	FRIDAY	SATURDAY	NOTES
3	4	5	_____
			_____
			_____
			_____
10	11	12	_____
			_____
			_____
			_____
17	18	19	_____
			_____
			_____
			_____
24	25	26	_____
			_____
			_____
CHRISTMAS EVE	CHRISTMAS DAY		_____
31			_____
			_____
			_____
NEW YEAR'S EVE			_____

✦ M O N • December, 30 2019

_____ ○ _____
_____ ○ _____
_____ ○ _____
_____ ○ _____
_____ ○ _____
_____ ○ _____
_____ ○ _____

✦ T U E • December 31, 2019

_____ ○ _____
_____ ○ _____
_____ ○ _____
_____ ○ _____
_____ ○ _____
_____ ○ _____
NEW YEAR'S EVE ____ ○ _____

✦ W E D • January 01, 2020

_____ ○ _____
_____ ○ _____
_____ ○ _____
_____ ○ _____
_____ ○ _____
_____ ○ _____
NEW YEAR'S DAY ____ ○ _____

✦ T H U • January 02, 2020

_____ ○ _____
_____ ○ _____
_____ ○ _____
_____ ○ _____
_____ ○ _____
_____ ○ _____
_____ ○ _____

FRI • January 03, 2020

_____   ○ _____
_____   ○ _____
_____   ○ _____
_____   ○ _____
_____   ○ _____
_____   ○ _____
_____   ○ _____

SAT • January 04, 2020

_____   ○ _____
_____   ○ _____
_____   ○ _____
_____   ○ _____
_____   ○ _____
_____   ○ _____
_____   ○ _____

SUN • January 05, 2020

_____   ○ _____
_____   ○ _____
_____   ○ _____
_____   ○ _____
_____   ○ _____
_____   ○ _____
_____   ○ _____

TO DO   ## NOTE

_____   ○ _____
_____   ○ _____
_____   ○ _____
_____   ○ _____
_____   ○ _____
_____   ○ _____
                            ○ _____

✦ M O N • January, 6 2020

_____   ○   _____
_____   ○   _____
_____   ○   _____
_____   ○   _____
_____   ○   _____
_____   ○   _____
_____   ○   _____

✦ T U E • January 07, 2020

_____   ○   _____
_____   ○   _____
_____   ○   _____
_____   ○   _____
_____   ○   _____
_____   ○   _____
_____   ○   _____

✦ W E D • January 08, 2020

_____   ○   _____
_____   ○   _____
_____   ○   _____
_____   ○   _____
_____   ○   _____
_____   ○   _____
_____   ○   _____

✦ T H U • January 09, 2020

_____   ○   _____
_____   ○   _____
_____   ○   _____
_____   ○   _____
_____   ○   _____
_____   ○   _____
_____   ○   _____

FRI • January 10, 2020

_____
_____
_____
_____
_____
_____

○ _____
○ _____
○ _____
○ _____
○ _____
○ _____
○ _____

SAT • January 11, 2020

_____
_____
_____
_____
_____
_____
_____

○ _____
○ _____
○ _____
○ _____
○ _____
○ _____
○ _____

SUN • January 12, 2020

_____
_____
_____
_____
_____
_____
_____

○ _____
○ _____
○ _____
○ _____
○ _____
○ _____
○ _____

TO DO

_____
_____
_____
_____
_____

NOTE

○ _____
○ _____
○ _____
○ _____
○ _____
○ _____
○ _____

◈ M O N • January, 13 2020

_____   ○
_____   ○ _____
_____   ○ _____
_____   ○ _____
_____   ○ _____
_____   ○ _____
_____   ○ _____
                              ○ _____

◈ T U E • January 14, 2020

_____   ○
_____   ○ _____
_____   ○ _____
_____   ○ _____
_____   ○ _____
_____   ○ _____
_____   ○ _____
                              ○ _____

◈ W E D • January 15, 2020

_____   ○
_____   ○ _____
_____   ○ _____
_____   ○ _____
_____   ○ _____
_____   ○ _____
_____   ○ _____
                              ○ _____

◈ T H U • January 16, 2020

_____   ○
_____   ○ _____
_____   ○ _____
_____   ○ _____
_____   ○ _____
_____   ○ _____
_____   ○ _____

FRI • January 17, 2020

_____   ○ _____
_____   ○ _____
_____   ○ _____
_____   ○ _____
_____   ○ _____
_____   ○ _____
_____   ○ _____

SAT • January 18, 2020

_____   ○ _____
_____   ○ _____
_____   ○ _____
_____   ○ _____
_____   ○ _____
_____   ○ _____
_____   ○ _____

SUN • January 19, 2020

_____   ○ _____
_____   ○ _____
_____   ○ _____
_____   ○ _____
_____   ○ _____
_____   ○ _____
_____   ○ _____

TO DO   ## NOTE

_____   ○ _____
_____   ○ _____
_____   ○ _____
_____   ○ _____
_____   ○ _____
                               ○ _____
                               ○ _____

❈ M O N • January, 20 2020

_____   ○
_____   ○ _____
_____   ○ _____
_____   ○ _____
_____   ○ _____
_____   ○ _____
MARTIN LUTHER KING JR. DAY   ○ _____
                                   _____

❈ T U E • January 21, 2020

                                ○ _____
_____   ○ _____
_____   ○ _____
_____   ○ _____
_____   ○ _____
_____   ○ _____
_____   ○ _____

❈ W E D • January 22, 2020

                                ○ _____
_____   ○ _____
_____   ○ _____
_____   ○ _____
_____   ○ _____
_____   ○ _____
_____   ○ _____

❈ T H U • January 23, 2020

                                ○ _____
_____   ○ _____
_____   ○ _____
_____   ○ _____
_____   ○ _____
_____   ○ _____
_____   ○ _____

❋ F R I • January 24, 2020

_____
_____
_____
_____
_____
_____

○ _____
○ _____
○ _____
○ _____
○ _____
○ _____
○ _____

❋ S A T • January 25, 2020

_____
_____
_____
_____
_____
_____

○ _____
○ _____
○ _____
○ _____
○ _____
○ _____
○ _____

❋ S U N • January 26, 2020

_____
_____
_____
_____
_____
_____

○ _____
○ _____
○ _____
○ _____
○ _____
○ _____
○ _____

TO DO

_____
_____
_____
_____

NOTE

○ _____
○ _____
○ _____
○ _____
○ _____
○ _____
○ _____

❖ M O N • January, 27 2020

_____
_____
_____
_____
_____
_____
_____

○ _____
○ _____
○ _____
○ _____
○ _____
○ _____
○ _____

❖ T U E • January 28, 2020

_____
_____
_____
_____
_____
_____
_____

○ _____
○ _____
○ _____
○ _____
○ _____
○ _____
○ _____

❖ W E D • January 29, 2020

_____
_____
_____
_____
_____
_____
_____

○ _____
○ _____
○ _____
○ _____
○ _____
○ _____
○ _____

❖ T H U • January 30, 2020

_____
_____
_____
_____
_____
_____
_____

○ _____
○ _____
○ _____
○ _____
○ _____
○ _____
○ _____

FRI • January 31, 2020

_____ ○ _____
_____ ○ _____
_____ ○ _____
_____ ○ _____
_____ ○ _____
_____ ○ _____
_____ ○ _____

SAT • February 01, 2020

_____ ○ _____
_____ ○ _____
_____ ○ _____
_____ ○ _____
_____ ○ _____
_____ ○ _____
_____ ○ _____

SUN • February 02, 2020

_____ ○ _____
_____ ○ _____
_____ ○ _____
_____ ○ _____
_____ ○ _____
_____ ○ _____
GROUNDHOG DAY   ○ _____

TO DO   ## NOTE

_____ ○ _____
_____ ○ _____
_____ ○ _____
_____ ○ _____
_____ ○ _____
_____ ○ _____
_____ ○ _____

MON • February, 3 2020

_____ ○ _____
_____ ○ _____
_____ ○ _____
_____ ○ _____
_____ ○ _____
_____ ○ _____
_____ ○ _____

TUE • February 04, 2020

_____ ○ _____
_____ ○ _____
_____ ○ _____
_____ ○ _____
_____ ○ _____
_____ ○ _____
_____ ○ _____

WED • February 05, 2020

_____ ○ _____
_____ ○ _____
_____ ○ _____
_____ ○ _____
_____ ○ _____
_____ ○ _____
_____ ○ _____

THU • February 06, 2020

_____ ○ _____
_____ ○ _____
_____ ○ _____
_____ ○ _____
_____ ○ _____
_____ ○ _____
_____ ○ _____

F   R   I • February 07, 2020

_____   ○ _____
_____   ○ _____
_____   ○ _____
_____   ○ _____
_____   ○ _____
_____   ○ _____
_____   ○ _____

S   A   T • February 08, 2020

_____   ○ _____
_____   ○ _____
_____   ○ _____
_____   ○ _____
_____   ○ _____
_____   ○ _____
_____   ○ _____

S   U   N • February 09, 2020

_____   ○ _____
_____   ○ _____
_____   ○ _____
_____   ○ _____
_____   ○ _____
_____   ○ _____
_____   ○ _____

TO DO   ## NOTE

_____   ○ _____
_____   ○ _____
_____   ○ _____
_____   ○ _____
_____   ○ _____
_____   ○ _____
_____   ○ _____

✦ M O N • February, 10 2020

_____
_____   ○   _____
_____   ○   _____
_____   ○   _____
_____   ○   _____
_____   ○   _____
_____   ○   _____
_____   ○

✦ T U E • February 11, 2020

_____   ○
_____   ○   _____
_____   ○   _____
_____   ○   _____
_____   ○   _____
_____   ○   _____
_____   ○   _____
_____   ○

✦ W E D • February 12, 2020

_____   ○
_____   ○   _____
_____   ○   _____
_____   ○   _____
_____   ○   _____
_____   ○   _____
_____   ○   _____
_____   ○

✦ T H U • February 13, 2020

_____   ○
_____   ○   _____
_____   ○   _____
_____   ○   _____
_____   ○   _____
_____   ○   _____
_____   ○   _____

❁ F R I • February 14, 2020

_____
_____   ○ _____
_____   ○ _____
_____   ○ _____
_____   ○ _____
_____   ○ _____
_____   ○ _____
VALENTINE'S DAY _____   ○ _____

❁ S A T • February 15, 2020

_____   ○ _____
_____   ○ _____
_____   ○ _____
_____   ○ _____
_____   ○ _____
_____   ○ _____
_____   ○ _____

❁ S U N • February 16, 2020

_____   ○ _____
_____   ○ _____
_____   ○ _____
_____   ○ _____
_____   ○ _____
_____   ○ _____
_____   ○ _____

TO DO   NOTE

_____   ○ _____
_____   ○ _____
_____   ○ _____
_____   ○ _____
_____   ○ _____
_____   ○ _____
_____   ○ _____

❖ M O N • February, 17 2020

_____   ◯   _____
_____   ◯   _____
_____   ◯   _____
_____   ◯   _____
_____   ◯   _____
_____   ◯   _____
PRESIDENTS' DAY   ◯   _____

❖ T U E • February 18, 2020

_____   ◯   _____
_____   ◯   _____
_____   ◯   _____
_____   ◯   _____
_____   ◯   _____
_____   ◯   _____
_____   ◯   _____

❖ W E D • February 19, 2020

_____   ◯   _____
_____   ◯   _____
_____   ◯   _____
_____   ◯   _____
_____   ◯   _____
_____   ◯   _____
_____   ◯   _____

❖ T H U • February 20, 2020

_____   ◯   _____
_____   ◯   _____
_____   ◯   _____
_____   ◯   _____
_____   ◯   _____
_____   ◯   _____
_____   ◯   _____

❖ F R I • February 21, 2020

_____   ○ _____
_____   ○ _____
_____   ○ _____
_____   ○ _____
_____   ○ _____
_____   ○ _____
_____   ○ _____

❖ S A T • February 22, 2020

_____   ○ _____
_____   ○ _____
_____   ○ _____
_____   ○ _____
_____   ○ _____
_____   ○ _____
_____   ○ _____

❖ S U N • February 23, 2020

_____   ○ _____
_____   ○ _____
_____   ○ _____
_____   ○ _____
_____   ○ _____
_____   ○ _____
_____   ○ _____

TO DO   ## NOTE

_____   ○ _____
_____   ○ _____
_____   ○ _____
_____   ○ _____
_____   ○ _____
_____   ○ _____
                                   ○ _____

❖ M O N • February, 24 2020

_____   ⭘   _____
_____   ⭘   _____
_____   ⭘   _____
_____   ⭘   _____
_____   ⭘   _____
_____   ⭘   _____
_____   ⭘   _____

❖ T U E • February 25, 2020

_____   ⭘   _____
_____   ⭘   _____
_____   ⭘   _____
_____   ⭘   _____
_____   ⭘   _____
_____   ⭘   _____
_____   ⭘   _____

❖ W E D • February 26, 2020

_____   ⭘   _____
_____   ⭘   _____
_____   ⭘   _____
_____   ⭘   _____
_____   ⭘   _____
_____   ⭘   _____
_____   ⭘   _____

❖ T H U • February 27, 2020

_____   ⭘   _____
_____   ⭘   _____
_____   ⭘   _____
_____   ⭘   _____
_____   ⭘   _____
_____   ⭘   _____
_____   ⭘   _____

❈ F   R   I • February 28, 2020

_____   ◯ _____
_____   ◯ _____
_____   ◯ _____
_____   ◯ _____
_____   ◯ _____
_____   ◯ _____
_____   ◯ _____

❈ S   A   T • February 29, 2020

_____   ◯ _____
_____   ◯ _____
_____   ◯ _____
_____   ◯ _____
_____   ◯ _____
_____   ◯ _____
_____   ◯ _____

❈ S   U   N • March 01, 2020

_____   ◯ _____
_____   ◯ _____
_____   ◯ _____
_____   ◯ _____
_____   ◯ _____
_____   ◯ _____
_____   ◯ _____

TO DO   NOTE

_____   ◯ _____
_____   ◯ _____
_____   ◯ _____
_____   ◯ _____
_____   ◯ _____
_____   ◯ _____
                                     ◯ _____

❖ M O N • March, 2 2020

_____   ◯ _____
_____   ◯ _____
_____   ◯ _____
_____   ◯ _____
_____   ◯ _____
_____   ◯ _____
_____   ◯ _____

❖ T U E • March 03, 2020

_____   ◯ _____
_____   ◯ _____
_____   ◯ _____
_____   ◯ _____
_____   ◯ _____
_____   ◯ _____
_____   ◯ _____

❖ W E D • March 04, 2020

_____   ◯ _____
_____   ◯ _____
_____   ◯ _____
_____   ◯ _____
_____   ◯ _____
_____   ◯ _____
_____   ◯ _____

❖ T H U • March 05, 2020

_____   ◯ _____
_____   ◯ _____
_____   ◯ _____
_____   ◯ _____
_____   ◯ _____
_____   ◯ _____
_____   ◯ _____

❀ F R I • March 06, 2020

_____   ○   _____
_____   ○   _____
_____   ○   _____
_____   ○   _____
_____   ○   _____
_____   ○   _____
_____   ○   _____

❀ S A T • March 07, 2020

_____   ○   _____
_____   ○   _____
_____   ○   _____
_____   ○   _____
_____   ○   _____
_____   ○   _____
_____   ○   _____

❀ S U N • March 08, 2020

_____   ○   _____
_____   ○   _____
_____   ○   _____
_____   ○   _____
_____   ○   _____
_____   ○   _____
_____   ○   _____

TO DO   ## NOTE

_____   ○   _____
_____   ○   _____
_____   ○   _____
_____   ○   _____
_____   ○   _____
_____   ○   _____
_____   ○   _____

✤ M O N • March, 9 2020

_____
_____ ○
_____ ○ _____
_____ ○ _____
_____ ○ _____
_____ ○ _____
_____ ○ _____
_____ ○ _____
                         ○ _____

✤ T U E • March 10, 2020

_____
_____ ○ _____
_____ ○ _____
_____ ○ _____
_____ ○ _____
_____ ○ _____
_____ ○ _____
                         ○ _____

✤ W E D • March 11, 2020

_____
_____ ○ _____
_____ ○ _____
_____ ○ _____
_____ ○ _____
_____ ○ _____
_____ ○ _____
                         ○ _____

✤ T H U • March 12, 2020

_____
_____ ○ _____
_____ ○ _____
_____ ○ _____
_____ ○ _____
_____ ○ _____
_____ ○ _____
                         ○ _____

FRI • March 13, 2020

_____ ○ _____
_____ ○ _____
_____ ○ _____
_____ ○ _____
_____ ○ _____
_____ ○ _____
_____ ○ _____

SAT • March 14, 2020

_____ ○ _____
_____ ○ _____
_____ ○ _____
_____ ○ _____
_____ ○ _____
_____ ○ _____
_____ ○ _____

SUN • March 15, 2020

_____ ○ _____
_____ ○ _____
_____ ○ _____
_____ ○ _____
_____ ○ _____
_____ ○ _____
_____ ○ _____

TO DO   ## NOTE

_____ ○ _____
_____ ○ _____
_____ ○ _____
_____ ○ _____
_____ ○ _____
_____ ○ _____
                          ○ _____

✦ M O N • March, 16 2020

_____ ◯ _____
_____ ◯ _____
_____ ◯ _____
_____ ◯ _____
_____ ◯ _____
_____ ◯ _____
_____ ◯ _____

✦ T U E • March 17, 2020

_____ ◯ _____
_____ ◯ _____
_____ ◯ _____
_____ ◯ _____
_____ ◯ _____
_____ ◯ _____
ST. PATRICK'S DAY   ◯ _____

✦ W E D • March 18, 2020

_____ ◯ _____
_____ ◯ _____
_____ ◯ _____
_____ ◯ _____
_____ ◯ _____
_____ ◯ _____
_____ ◯ _____

✦ T H U • March 19, 2020

_____ ◯ _____
_____ ◯ _____
_____ ◯ _____
_____ ◯ _____
_____ ◯ _____
_____ ◯ _____
_____ ◯ _____

❈ F R I • March 20, 2020

_____
_____
_____
_____
_____
_____

○ _____
○ _____
○ _____
○ _____
○ _____
○ _____
○ _____

❈ S A T • March 21, 2020

_____
_____
_____
_____
_____
_____
_____
_____

○ _____
○ _____
○ _____
○ _____
○ _____
○ _____
○ _____

❈ S U N • March 22, 2020

_____
_____
_____
_____
_____
_____
_____

○ _____
○ _____
○ _____
○ _____
○ _____
○ _____
○ _____

TO DO

_____
_____
_____
_____
_____

NOTE

○ _____
○ _____
○ _____
○ _____
○ _____
○ _____
○ _____

MON • March, 23 2020

_____   ○   _____
_____   ○   _____
_____   ○   _____
_____   ○   _____
_____   ○   _____
_____   ○   _____
_____   ○   _____

TUE • March 24, 2020

_____   ○   _____
_____   ○   _____
_____   ○   _____
_____   ○   _____
_____   ○   _____
_____   ○   _____
_____   ○   _____

WED • March 25, 2020

_____   ○   _____
_____   ○   _____
_____   ○   _____
_____   ○   _____
_____   ○   _____
_____   ○   _____
_____   ○   _____

THU • March 26, 2020

_____   ○   _____
_____   ○   _____
_____   ○   _____
_____   ○   _____
_____   ○   _____
_____   ○   _____
_____   ○   _____

✦ F R I • March 27, 2020

_____
_____
_____
_____
_____
_____

○ _____
○ _____
○ _____
○ _____
○ _____
○ _____
○ _____

✦ S A T • March 28, 2020

_____
_____
_____
_____
_____
_____
_____
_____
_____

○ _____
○ _____
○ _____
○ _____
○ _____
○ _____
○ _____

✦ S U N • March 29, 2020

_____
_____
_____
_____
_____
_____
_____
_____
_____

○ _____
○ _____
○ _____
○ _____
○ _____
○ _____
○ _____

TO DO

_____
_____
_____
_____
_____
_____

NOTE

○ _____
○ _____
○ _____
○ _____
○ _____
○ _____
○ _____

✦ M O N • March, 30 2020

_____ ⃝ _____
_____ ⃝ _____
_____ ⃝ _____
_____ ⃝ _____
_____ ⃝ _____
_____ ⃝ _____
_____ ⃝ _____

✦ T U E • March 31, 2020

_____ ⃝ _____
_____ ⃝ _____
_____ ⃝ _____
_____ ⃝ _____
_____ ⃝ _____
_____ ⃝ _____
_____ ⃝ _____

✦ W E D • April 01, 2020

_____ ⃝ _____
_____ ⃝ _____
_____ ⃝ _____
_____ ⃝ _____
_____ ⃝ _____
_____ ⃝ _____
_____ ⃝ _____

✦ T H U • April 02, 2020

_____ ⃝ _____
_____ ⃝ _____
_____ ⃝ _____
_____ ⃝ _____
_____ ⃝ _____
_____ ⃝ _____
_____ ⃝ _____

✤ F R I • April 03, 2020

_____ ○ _____
_____ ○ _____
_____ ○ _____
_____ ○ _____
_____ ○ _____
_____ ○ _____
_____ ○ _____

✤ S A T • April 04, 2020

_____ ○ _____
_____ ○ _____
_____ ○ _____
_____ ○ _____
_____ ○ _____
_____ ○ _____
_____ ○ _____

✤ S U N • April 05, 2020

_____ ○ _____
_____ ○ _____
_____ ○ _____
_____ ○ _____
_____ ○ _____
_____ ○ _____
_____ ○ _____

TO DO

_____
_____
_____
_____
_____

NOTE

○ _____
○ _____
○ _____
○ _____
○ _____
○ _____
○ _____

✽ M O N • April, 6 2020

_____   ⃝ _____
_____   ⃝ _____
_____   ⃝ _____
_____   ⃝ _____
_____   ⃝ _____
_____   ⃝ _____
_____   ⃝ _____

✽ T U E • April 07, 2020

_____   ⃝ _____
_____   ⃝ _____
_____   ⃝ _____
_____   ⃝ _____
_____   ⃝ _____
_____   ⃝ _____
_____   ⃝ _____

✽ W E D • April 08, 2020

_____   ⃝ _____
_____   ⃝ _____
_____   ⃝ _____
_____   ⃝ _____
_____   ⃝ _____
_____   ⃝ _____
_____   ⃝ _____

✽ T H U • April 09, 2020

_____   ⃝ _____
_____   ⃝ _____
_____   ⃝ _____
_____   ⃝ _____
_____   ⃝ _____
_____   ⃝ _____
_____   ⃝ _____

❖ F R I • April 10, 2020

_____   ◯
_____   ◯   _____
_____   ◯   _____
_____   ◯   _____
_____   ◯   _____
_____   ◯   _____
_____   ◯   _____
                             ◯   _____

❖ S A T • April 11, 2020

_____   ◯   _____
_____   ◯   _____
_____   ◯   _____
_____   ◯   _____
_____   ◯   _____
_____   ◯   _____
_____   ◯   _____

❖ S U N • April 12, 2020

_____   ◯   _____
_____   ◯   _____
_____   ◯   _____
_____   ◯   _____
_____   ◯   _____
_____   ◯   _____
EASTER DAY   ◯   _____

TO DO   # NOTE

_____   ◯   _____
_____   ◯   _____
_____   ◯   _____
_____   ◯   _____
_____   ◯   _____
_____   ◯   _____
_____   ◯   _____

✧ M O N • April, 13 2020

_____   ◯
_____   ◯   _____
_____   ◯   _____
_____   ◯   _____
_____   ◯   _____
_____   ◯   _____
_____   ◯   _____
                            ◯   _____

✧ T U E • April 14, 2020

_____   ◯
_____   ◯   _____
_____   ◯   _____
_____   ◯   _____
_____   ◯   _____
_____   ◯   _____
_____   ◯   _____

✧ W E D • April 15, 2020

_____   ◯
_____   ◯   _____
_____   ◯   _____
_____   ◯   _____
_____   ◯   _____
_____   ◯   _____
TAX DAY   ◯   _____

✧ T H U • April 16, 2020

_____   ◯
_____   ◯   _____
_____   ◯   _____
_____   ◯   _____
_____   ◯   _____
_____   ◯   _____
_____   ◯   _____

FRI • April 17, 2020

○
○
○
○
○
○
○

SAT • April 18, 2020

○
○
○
○
○
○
○

SUN • April 19, 2020

○
○
○
○
○
○
○

TO DO

NOTE

○
○
○
○
○
○
○

✤ M O N • April, 20 2020

_____ ⭘ _____
_____ ⭘ _____
_____ ⭘ _____
_____ ⭘ _____
_____ ⭘ _____
_____ ⭘ _____
_____ ⭘ _____

✤ T U E • April 21, 2020

_____ ⭘ _____
_____ ⭘ _____
_____ ⭘ _____
_____ ⭘ _____
_____ ⭘ _____
_____ ⭘ _____
_____ ⭘ _____

✤ W E D • April 22, 2020

_____ ⭘ _____
_____ ⭘ _____
_____ ⭘ _____
_____ ⭘ _____
_____ ⭘ _____
_____ ⭘ _____
_____ ⭘ _____

✤ T H U • April 23, 2020

_____ ⭘ _____
_____ ⭘ _____
_____ ⭘ _____
_____ ⭘ _____
_____ ⭘ _____
_____ ⭘ _____
_____ ⭘ _____

❀ F R I • April 24, 2020

_____   ○
_____   ○ _____
_____   ○ _____
_____   ○ _____
_____   ○ _____
_____   ○ _____
_____   ○ _____
                              ○ _____

❀ S A T • April 25, 2020

                              ○ _____
_____   ○ _____
_____   ○ _____
_____   ○ _____
_____   ○ _____
_____   ○ _____
_____   ○ _____
_____   ○

❀ S U N • April 26, 2020

                              ○ _____
_____   ○ _____
_____   ○ _____
_____   ○ _____
_____   ○ _____
_____   ○ _____
_____   ○ _____
_____   ○

TO DO   NOTE

                              ○
_____   ○ _____
_____   ○ _____
_____   ○ _____
_____   ○ _____
_____   ○ _____
_____   ○ _____
_____   ○ _____

❈ M O N • April, 27 2020

_____
_____   ◯
_____   ◯
_____   ◯
_____   ◯   _____
_____   ◯   _____
_____   ◯   _____
                             ◯   _____
                                   _____

❈ T U E • April 28, 2020

_____   ◯
_____   ◯
_____   ◯   _____
_____   ◯   _____
_____   ◯   _____
_____   ◯   _____
_____   ◯   _____

❈ W E D • April 29, 2020

_____   ◯
_____   ◯
_____   ◯   _____
_____   ◯   _____
_____   ◯   _____
_____   ◯   _____
_____   ◯   _____

❈ T H U • April 30, 2020

_____   ◯
_____   ◯
_____   ◯   _____
_____   ◯   _____
_____   ◯   _____
_____   ◯   _____
_____   ◯   _____

❀ F   R   I • May 01, 2020

_____ ○ _____
_____ ○ _____
_____ ○ _____
_____ ○ _____
_____ ○ _____
_____ ○ _____
_____ ○ _____

❀ S   A   T • May 02, 2020

_____ ○ _____
_____ ○ _____
_____ ○ _____
_____ ○ _____
_____ ○ _____
_____ ○ _____
_____ ○ _____

❀ S   U   N • May 03, 2020

_____ ○ _____
_____ ○ _____
_____ ○ _____
_____ ○ _____
_____ ○ _____
_____ ○ _____
_____ ○ _____

TO DO   ## NOTE

_____ ○ _____
_____ ○ _____
_____ ○ _____
_____ ○ _____
_____ ○ _____
_____ ○ _____
_____ ○ _____

❀ M O N • May, 4 2020

_____   ◯ _____
_____   ◯ _____
_____   ◯ _____
_____   ◯ _____
_____   ◯ _____
_____   ◯ _____
_____   ◯ _____

❀ T U E • May 05, 2020

_____   ◯ _____
_____   ◯ _____
_____   ◯ _____
_____   ◯ _____
_____   ◯ _____
_____   ◯ _____
CINCO DE MAYO   ◯ _____

❀ W E D • May 06, 2020

_____   ◯ _____
_____   ◯ _____
_____   ◯ _____
_____   ◯ _____
_____   ◯ _____
_____   ◯ _____
_____   ◯ _____

❀ T H U • May 07, 2020

_____   ◯ _____
_____   ◯ _____
_____   ◯ _____
_____   ◯ _____
_____   ◯ _____
_____   ◯ _____
_____   ◯ _____

✦ F R I • May 08, 2020

_____   ◯ _____
_____   ◯ _____
_____   ◯ _____
_____   ◯ _____
_____   ◯ _____
_____   ◯ _____
_____   ◯ _____

✦ S A T • May 09, 2020

_____   ◯ _____
_____   ◯ _____
_____   ◯ _____
_____   ◯ _____
_____   ◯ _____
_____   ◯ _____
_____   ◯ _____

✦ S U N • May 10, 2020

_____   ◯ _____
_____   ◯ _____
_____   ◯ _____
_____   ◯ _____
_____   ◯ _____
_____   ◯ _____
MOTHER'S DAY   ◯ _____

TO DO   # NOTE

_____   ◯ _____
_____   ◯ _____
_____   ◯ _____
_____   ◯ _____
_____   ◯ _____
_____   ◯ _____
                          ◯ _____

MON • May, 11 2020

_____ ○
_____ ○ _____
_____ ○ _____
_____ ○ _____
_____ ○ _____
_____ ○ _____
_____ ○ _____
                         ○ _____

TUE • May 12, 2020

_____ ○
_____ ○ _____
_____ ○ _____
_____ ○ _____
_____ ○ _____
_____ ○ _____
_____ ○ _____
                         ○ _____

WED • May 13, 2020

_____ ○
_____ ○ _____
_____ ○ _____
_____ ○ _____
_____ ○ _____
_____ ○ _____
_____ ○ _____
                         ○ _____

THU • May 14, 2020

_____ ○
_____ ○ _____
_____ ○ _____
_____ ○ _____
_____ ○ _____
_____ ○ _____
_____ ○ _____
                         ○ _____

F R I • May 15, 2020

_____ ○ _____
_____ ○ _____
_____ ○ _____
_____ ○ _____
_____ ○ _____
_____ ○ _____
_____ ○ _____

S A T • May 16, 2020

_____ ○ _____
_____ ○ _____
_____ ○ _____
_____ ○ _____
_____ ○ _____
_____ ○ _____
_____ ○ _____

S U N • May 17, 2020

_____ ○ _____
_____ ○ _____
_____ ○ _____
_____ ○ _____
_____ ○ _____
_____ ○ _____
_____ ○ _____

TO DO

NOTE

_____ ○ _____
_____ ○ _____
_____ ○ _____
_____ ○ _____
_____ ○ _____
_____ ○ _____
_____ ○ _____

❋ M O N • May, 18 2020

_____ ○ _____
_____ ○ _____
_____ ○ _____
_____ ○ _____
_____ ○ _____
_____ ○ _____
_____ ○ _____

❋ T U E • May 19, 2020

_____ ○ _____
_____ ○ _____
_____ ○ _____
_____ ○ _____
_____ ○ _____
_____ ○ _____
_____ ○ _____

❋ W E D • May 20, 2020

_____ ○ _____
_____ ○ _____
_____ ○ _____
_____ ○ _____
_____ ○ _____
_____ ○ _____
_____ ○ _____

❋ T H U • May 21, 2020

_____ ○ _____
_____ ○ _____
_____ ○ _____
_____ ○ _____
_____ ○ _____
_____ ○ _____
_____ ○ _____

FRI • May 22, 2020

_____   ○   _____
_____   ○   _____
_____   ○   _____
_____   ○   _____
_____   ○   _____
_____   ○   _____
_____   ○   _____

SAT • May 23, 2020

_____   ○   _____
_____   ○   _____
_____   ○   _____
_____   ○   _____
_____   ○   _____
_____   ○   _____
_____   ○   _____

SUN • May 24, 2020

_____   ○   _____
_____   ○   _____
_____   ○   _____
_____   ○   _____
_____   ○   _____
_____   ○   _____
_____   ○   _____

TO DO   ## NOTE

_____   ○   _____
_____   ○   _____
_____   ○   _____
_____   ○   _____
_____   ○   _____
_____   ○   _____
_____   ○   _____

❖ M O N • May, 25 2020

_____
_____
_____
_____
_____
_____
MEMORIAL DAY

○
○
○
○
○
○
○

_____
_____
_____
_____
_____
_____
_____

❖ T U E • May 26, 2020

_____
_____
_____
_____
_____
_____
_____

○
○
○
○
○
○
○

_____
_____
_____
_____
_____
_____
_____

❖ W E D • May 27, 2020

_____
_____
_____
_____
_____
_____
_____

○
○
○
○
○
○
○

_____
_____
_____
_____
_____
_____
_____

❖ T H U • May 28, 2020

_____
_____
_____
_____
_____
_____
_____

○
○
○
○
○
○
○

_____
_____
_____
_____
_____
_____
_____

FRI • May 29, 2020

_____
_____
_____
_____
_____
_____
_____

○ _____
○ _____
○ _____
○ _____
○ _____
○ _____
○ _____

SAT • May 30, 2020

_____
_____
_____
_____
_____
_____
_____

○ _____
○ _____
○ _____
○ _____
○ _____
○ _____
○ _____

SUN • May 31, 2020

_____
_____
_____
_____
_____
_____
_____

○ _____
○ _____
○ _____
○ _____
○ _____
○ _____
○ _____

TO DO

_____
_____
_____
_____
_____

NOTE

○ _____
○ _____
○ _____
○ _____
○ _____
○ _____
○ _____

❖ M O N • June, 1 2020

_____ ◯
_____ ◯ _____
_____ ◯ _____
_____ ◯ _____
_____ ◯ _____
_____ ◯ _____
_____ ◯ _____
                          ◯ _____

❖ T U E • June 02, 2020

_____ ◯
_____ ◯ _____
_____ ◯ _____
_____ ◯ _____
_____ ◯ _____
_____ ◯ _____
_____ ◯ _____
                          ◯ _____

❖ W E D • June 03, 2020

_____ ◯
_____ ◯ _____
_____ ◯ _____
_____ ◯ _____
_____ ◯ _____
_____ ◯ _____
_____ ◯ _____
                          ◯ _____

❖ T H U • June 04, 2020

_____ ◯
_____ ◯ _____
_____ ◯ _____
_____ ◯ _____
_____ ◯ _____
_____ ◯ _____
_____ ◯ _____
                          ◯ _____

FRI • June 05, 2020

_____ ○
_____ ○ _____
_____ ○ _____
_____ ○ _____
_____ ○ _____
_____ ○ _____
_____ ○ _____
                          ○ _____

SAT • June 06, 2020

_____ ○
_____ ○ _____
_____ ○ _____
_____ ○ _____
_____ ○ _____
_____ ○ _____
_____ ○ _____
                          ○ _____

SUN • June 07, 2020

_____ ○
_____ ○ _____
_____ ○ _____
_____ ○ _____
_____ ○ _____
_____ ○ _____
_____ ○ _____
                          ○ _____

TO DO   ## NOTE

_____ ○
_____ ○ _____
_____ ○ _____
_____ ○ _____
_____ ○ _____
_____ ○ _____
_____ ○ _____

❀ M O N • June, 8 2020

_____
_____
_____
_____
_____
_____
_____

○ _____
○ _____
○ _____
○ _____
○ _____
○ _____
○ _____

❀ T U E • June 09, 2020

_____
_____
_____
_____
_____
_____
_____

○ _____
○ _____
○ _____
○ _____
○ _____
○ _____
○ _____

❀ W E D • June 10, 2020

_____
_____
_____
_____
_____
_____
_____

○ _____
○ _____
○ _____
○ _____
○ _____
○ _____
○ _____

❀ T H U • June 11, 2020

_____
_____
_____
_____
_____
_____
_____

○ _____
○ _____
○ _____
○ _____
○ _____
○ _____
○ _____

�֎ F R I • June 12, 2020

_____
_____
_____
_____
_____
_____
_____

○ _____
○ _____
○ _____
○ _____
○ _____
○ _____
○ _____

✖ S A T • June 13, 2020

_____
_____
_____
_____
_____
_____
_____

○ _____
○ _____
○ _____
○ _____
○ _____
○ _____
○ _____

✖ S U N • June 14, 2020

_____
_____
_____
_____
_____
_____
_____

○ _____
○ _____
○ _____
○ _____
○ _____
○ _____
○ _____

TO DO

_____
_____
_____
_____
_____
_____

NOTE

○ _____
○ _____
○ _____
○ _____
○ _____
○ _____
○ _____

✦ M O N • June, 15 2020

_____
_____   ○
_____   ○   _____
_____   ○   _____
_____   ○   _____
_____   ○   _____
_____   ○   _____
                               ○   _____
                               ○   _____

✦ T U E • June 16, 2020

_____
_____   ○   _____
_____   ○   _____
_____   ○   _____
_____   ○   _____
_____   ○   _____
_____   ○   _____
                               ○   _____

✦ W E D • June 17, 2020

_____
_____   ○   _____
_____   ○   _____
_____   ○   _____
_____   ○   _____
_____   ○   _____
_____   ○   _____
                               ○   _____

✦ T H U • June 18, 2020

_____
_____   ○   _____
_____   ○   _____
_____   ○   _____
_____   ○   _____
_____   ○   _____
_____   ○   _____
                               ○   _____

✤ F R I • June 19, 2020

○
○
○
○
○
○
○

✤ S A T • June 20, 2020

○
○
○
○
○
○
○

✤ S U N • June 21, 2020

FATHER'S DAY

○
○
○
○
○
○
○

TO DO

NOTE

○
○
○
○
○
○
○

❖ M O N • June, 22 2020

_____
_____   ◯ _____
_____   ◯ _____
_____   ◯ _____
_____   ◯ _____
_____   ◯ _____
_____   ◯ _____
                                          ◯ _____

❖ T U E • June 23, 2020

_____
_____   ◯ _____
_____   ◯ _____
_____   ◯ _____
_____   ◯ _____
_____   ◯ _____
_____   ◯ _____
                                          ◯ _____

❖ W E D • June 24, 2020

_____
_____   ◯ _____
_____   ◯ _____
_____   ◯ _____
_____   ◯ _____
_____   ◯ _____
_____   ◯ _____
                                          ◯ _____

❖ T H U • June 25, 2020

_____
_____   ◯ _____
_____   ◯ _____
_____   ◯ _____
_____   ◯ _____
_____   ◯ _____
_____   ◯ _____
                                          ◯ _____

F R I • June 26, 2020

_____ ○
_____ ○ _____
_____ ○ _____
_____ ○ _____
_____ ○ _____
_____ ○ _____
_____ ○ _____
                         ○ _____

S A T • June 27, 2020

_____ ○
_____ ○ _____
_____ ○ _____
_____ ○ _____
_____ ○ _____
_____ ○ _____
_____ ○ _____
_____ ○ _____

S U N • June 28, 2020

_____ ○
_____ ○ _____
_____ ○ _____
_____ ○ _____
_____ ○ _____
_____ ○ _____
_____ ○ _____

TO DO   ## NOTE

_____ ○
_____ ○ _____
_____ ○ _____
_____ ○ _____
_____ ○ _____
_____ ○ _____
_____ ○ _____

MON • June, 29 2020

_____   ○   _____
_____   ○   _____
_____   ○   _____
_____   ○   _____
_____   ○   _____
_____   ○   _____
_____   ○   _____

TUE • June 30, 2020

_____   ○   _____
_____   ○   _____
_____   ○   _____
_____   ○   _____
_____   ○   _____
_____   ○   _____
_____   ○   _____

WED • July 01, 2020

_____   ○   _____
_____   ○   _____
_____   ○   _____
_____   ○   _____
_____   ○   _____
_____   ○   _____
_____   ○   _____

THU • July 02, 2020

_____   ○   _____
_____   ○   _____
_____   ○   _____
_____   ○   _____
_____   ○   _____
_____   ○   _____
_____   ○   _____

✤ F R I • July 03, 2020

_____
_____
_____
_____
_____
_____
INDEPENDENCE DAY (OBSERVED)

○ _____
○ _____
○ _____
○ _____
○ _____
○ _____
○ _____

✤ S A T • July 04, 2020

_____
_____
_____
_____
_____
_____
INDEPENDENCE DAY

○ _____
○ _____
○ _____
○ _____
○ _____
○ _____
○ _____

✤ S U N • July 05, 2020

_____
_____
_____
_____
_____
_____
_____

○ _____
○ _____
○ _____
○ _____
○ _____
○ _____
○ _____

TO DO

_____
_____
_____
_____
_____
_____

NOTE

○ _____
○ _____
○ _____
○ _____
○ _____
○ _____
○ _____

✤ M O N • July, 6 2020

_____
_____
_____
_____
_____
_____

○ _____
○ _____
○ _____
○ _____
○ _____
○ _____
○ _____

✤ T U E • July 07, 2020

_____
_____
_____
_____
_____
_____
_____

○ _____
○ _____
○ _____
○ _____
○ _____
○ _____
○ _____

✤ W E D • July 08, 2020

_____
_____
_____
_____
_____
_____

○ _____
○ _____
○ _____
○ _____
○ _____
○ _____
○ _____

✤ T H U • July 09, 2020

_____
_____
_____
_____
_____

○ _____
○ _____
○ _____
○ _____
○ _____
○ _____
○ _____

❈ F R I • July 10, 2020

_____
_____   ⭕ _____
_____   ⭕ _____
_____   ⭕ _____
_____   ⭕ _____
_____   ⭕ _____
_____   ⭕ _____
                          ⭕ _____
                          ⭕ _____

❈ S A T • July 11, 2020

_____
_____   ⭕ _____
_____   ⭕ _____
_____   ⭕ _____
_____   ⭕ _____
_____   ⭕ _____
_____   ⭕ _____
_____   ⭕ _____

❈ S U N • July 12, 2020

_____   ⭕ _____
_____   ⭕ _____
_____   ⭕ _____
_____   ⭕ _____
_____   ⭕ _____
_____   ⭕ _____
_____   ⭕ _____

TO DO   ## NOTE

_____   ⭕ _____
_____   ⭕ _____
_____   ⭕ _____
_____   ⭕ _____
_____   ⭕ _____
_____   ⭕ _____
                          ⭕ _____

M O N • July, 13 2020

_____ ○ _____
_____ ○ _____
_____ ○ _____
_____ ○ _____
_____ ○ _____
_____ ○ _____
_____ ○ _____

T U E • July 14, 2020

_____ ○ _____
_____ ○ _____
_____ ○ _____
_____ ○ _____
_____ ○ _____
_____ ○ _____
_____ ○ _____

W E D • July 15, 2020

_____ ○ _____
_____ ○ _____
_____ ○ _____
_____ ○ _____
_____ ○ _____
_____ ○ _____
_____ ○ _____

T H U • July 16, 2020

_____ ○ _____
_____ ○ _____
_____ ○ _____
_____ ○ _____
_____ ○ _____
_____ ○ _____
_____ ○ _____

F R I • July 17, 2020

○
○
○
○
○
○
○

S A T • July 18, 2020

○
○
○
○
○
○
○

S U N • July 19, 2020

○
○
○
○
○
○
○

TO DO

NOTE

○
○
○
○
○
○
○

✦ M O N • July, 20 2020

_____
_____
_____
_____
_____
_____
_____

○ _____
○ _____
○ _____
○ _____
○ _____
○ _____
○ _____

✦ T U E • July 21, 2020

_____
_____
_____
_____
_____
_____
_____

○ _____
○ _____
○ _____
○ _____
○ _____
○ _____
○ _____

✦ W E D • July 22, 2020

_____
_____
_____
_____
_____
_____
_____

○ _____
○ _____
○ _____
○ _____
○ _____
○ _____
○ _____

✦ T H U • July 23, 2020

_____
_____
_____
_____
_____
_____
_____

○ _____
○ _____
○ _____
○ _____
○ _____
○ _____
○ _____

�֎ F R I • July 24, 2020

_____ ◯ _____
_____ ◯ _____
_____ ◯ _____
_____ ◯ _____
_____ ◯ _____
_____ ◯ _____
_____ ◯ _____

�֎ S A T • July 25, 2020

_____ ◯ _____
_____ ◯ _____
_____ ◯ _____
_____ ◯ _____
_____ ◯ _____
_____ ◯ _____
_____ ◯ _____

✖ S U N • July 26, 2020

_____ ◯ _____
_____ ◯ _____
_____ ◯ _____
_____ ◯ _____
_____ ◯ _____
_____ ◯ _____
_____ ◯ _____

TO DO   ## NOTE

_____ ◯ _____
_____ ◯ _____
_____ ◯ _____
_____ ◯ _____
_____ ◯ _____
_____ ◯ _____
_____ ◯ _____

MON • July, 27 2020

_____   ○
_____   ○   _____
_____   ○   _____
_____   ○   _____
_____   ○   _____
_____   ○   _____
_____   ○   _____
                           ○   _____

TUE • July 28, 2020

_____   ○
_____   ○   _____
_____   ○   _____
_____   ○   _____
_____   ○   _____
_____   ○   _____
_____   ○   _____
                           ○   _____

WED • July 29, 2020

_____   ○
_____   ○   _____
_____   ○   _____
_____   ○   _____
_____   ○   _____
_____   ○   _____
_____   ○   _____
                           ○   _____

THU • July 30, 2020

_____   ○
_____   ○   _____
_____   ○   _____
_____   ○   _____
_____   ○   _____
_____   ○   _____
_____   ○   _____
                           ○   _____

FRI • July 31, 2020

_____   ○ _____
_____   ○ _____
_____   ○ _____
_____   ○ _____
_____   ○ _____
_____   ○ _____
_____   ○ _____

SAT • August 01, 2020

_____   ○ _____
_____   ○ _____
_____   ○ _____
_____   ○ _____
_____   ○ _____
_____   ○ _____
_____   ○ _____

SUN • August 02, 2020

_____   ○ _____
_____   ○ _____
_____   ○ _____
_____   ○ _____
_____   ○ _____
_____   ○ _____
_____   ○ _____

TO DO   # NOTE

_____   ○ _____
_____   ○ _____
_____   ○ _____
_____   ○ _____
_____   ○ _____
_____   ○ _____
_____   ○ _____

❖ M O N • August, 3 2020

_____ ◯ _____
_____ ◯ _____
_____ ◯ _____
_____ ◯ _____
_____ ◯ _____
_____ ◯ _____
_____ ◯ _____
_____ ◯ _____

❖ T U E • August 04, 2020

_____ ◯ _____
_____ ◯ _____
_____ ◯ _____
_____ ◯ _____
_____ ◯ _____
_____ ◯ _____
_____ ◯ _____

❖ W E D • August 05, 2020

_____ ◯ _____
_____ ◯ _____
_____ ◯ _____
_____ ◯ _____
_____ ◯ _____
_____ ◯ _____
_____ ◯ _____

❖ T H U • August 06, 2020

_____ ◯ _____
_____ ◯ _____
_____ ◯ _____
_____ ◯ _____
_____ ◯ _____
_____ ◯ _____
_____ ◯ _____

❖ F R I • August 07, 2020

_____ ○ _____
_____ ○ _____
_____ ○ _____
_____ ○ _____
_____ ○ _____
_____ ○ _____
_____ ○ _____

❖ S A T • August 08, 2020

_____ ○ _____
_____ ○ _____
_____ ○ _____
_____ ○ _____
_____ ○ _____
_____ ○ _____
_____ ○ _____

❖ S U N • August 09, 2020

_____ ○ _____
_____ ○ _____
_____ ○ _____
_____ ○ _____
_____ ○ _____
_____ ○ _____
_____ ○ _____

TO DO   ## NOTE

_____ ○ _____
_____ ○ _____
_____ ○ _____
_____ ○ _____
_____ ○ _____
_____ ○ _____
                            ○ _____

�҈ M O N • August, 10 2020

_____   ◯ _____
_____   ◯ _____
_____   ◯ _____
_____   ◯ _____
_____   ◯ _____
_____   ◯ _____
_____   ◯ _____

✲ T U E • August 11, 2020

_____   ◯ _____
_____   ◯ _____
_____   ◯ _____
_____   ◯ _____
_____   ◯ _____
_____   ◯ _____
_____   ◯ _____

✲ W E D • August 12, 2020

_____   ◯ _____
_____   ◯ _____
_____   ◯ _____
_____   ◯ _____
_____   ◯ _____
_____   ◯ _____
_____   ◯ _____

✲ T H U • August 13, 2020

_____   ◯ _____
_____   ◯ _____
_____   ◯ _____
_____   ◯ _____
_____   ◯ _____
_____   ◯ _____
_____   ◯ _____

❀ F R I • August 14, 2020

○
○
○
○
○
○
○

❀ S A T • August 15, 2020

○
○
○
○
○
○
○

❀ S U N • August 16, 2020

○
○
○
○
○
○
○

TO DO

NOTE

○
○
○
○
○
○
○

✾ M O N • August, 17 2020

_____
_____   ○ _____
_____   ○ _____
_____   ○ _____
_____   ○ _____
_____   ○ _____
_____   ○ _____
                                    ○ _____

✾ T U E • August 18, 2020

_____   ○ _____
_____   ○ _____
_____   ○ _____
_____   ○ _____
_____   ○ _____
_____   ○ _____
_____   ○ _____

✾ W E D • August 19, 2020

_____   ○ _____
_____   ○ _____
_____   ○ _____
_____   ○ _____
_____   ○ _____
_____   ○ _____
_____   ○ _____

✾ T H U • August 20, 2020

_____   ○ _____
_____   ○ _____
_____   ○ _____
_____   ○ _____
_____   ○ _____
_____   ○ _____
_____   ○ _____

❖ F R I • August 21, 2020

_____
_____
_____
_____
_____
_____
_____

○ _____
○ _____
○ _____
○ _____
○ _____
○ _____
○ _____

❖ S A T • August 22, 2020

_____
_____
_____
_____
_____
_____
_____

○ _____
○ _____
○ _____
○ _____
○ _____
○ _____
○ _____

❖ S U N • August 23, 2020

_____
_____
_____
_____
_____
_____
_____

○ _____
○ _____
○ _____
○ _____
○ _____
○ _____
○ _____

TO DO

_____
_____
_____
_____
_____

NOTE

○ _____
○ _____
○ _____
○ _____
○ _____
○ _____
○ _____

❖ M O N • August, 24 2020

_____ ○ _____
_____ ○ _____
_____ ○ _____
_____ ○ _____
_____ ○ _____
_____ ○ _____
_____ ○ _____

❖ T U   E • August 25, 2020

_____ ○ _____
_____ ○ _____
_____ ○ _____
_____ ○ _____
_____ ○ _____
_____ ○ _____
_____ ○ _____

❖ W E D • August 26, 2020

_____ ○ _____
_____ ○ _____
_____ ○ _____
_____ ○ _____
_____ ○ _____
_____ ○ _____
_____ ○ _____

❖ T H U • August 27, 2020

_____ ○ _____
_____ ○ _____
_____ ○ _____
_____ ○ _____
_____ ○ _____
_____ ○ _____
_____ ○ _____

F R I • August 28, 2020

_____   ○ _____
_____   ○ _____
_____   ○ _____
_____   ○ _____
_____   ○ _____
_____   ○ _____
_____   ○ _____

S A T • August 29, 2020

_____   ○ _____
_____   ○ _____
_____   ○ _____
_____   ○ _____
_____   ○ _____
_____   ○ _____
_____   ○ _____

S U N • August 30, 2020

_____   ○ _____
_____   ○ _____
_____   ○ _____
_____   ○ _____
_____   ○ _____
_____   ○ _____
_____   ○ _____

TO DO   ## NOTE

_____   ○ _____
_____   ○ _____
_____   ○ _____
_____   ○ _____
_____   ○ _____
_____   ○ _____
                            ○ _____

❖ M O N • August, 31 2020

_____   ○ _____
_____   ○ _____
_____   ○ _____
_____   ○ _____
_____   ○ _____
_____   ○ _____
_____   ○ _____

❖ T U E • September 01, 2020

_____   ○ _____
_____   ○ _____
_____   ○ _____
_____   ○ _____
_____   ○ _____
_____   ○ _____
_____   ○ _____

❖ W E D • September 02, 2020

_____   ○ _____
_____   ○ _____
_____   ○ _____
_____   ○ _____
_____   ○ _____
_____   ○ _____
_____   ○ _____

❖ T H U • September 03, 2020

_____   ○ _____
_____   ○ _____
_____   ○ _____
_____   ○ _____
_____   ○ _____
_____   ○ _____
_____   ○ _____

✥ F R I • September 04, 2020

_____
_____
_____
_____
_____
_____

○ _____
○ _____
○ _____
○ _____
○ _____
○ _____
○ _____
○ _____

✥ S A T • September 05, 2020

_____
_____
_____
_____
_____
_____
_____
_____

○ _____
○ _____
○ _____
○ _____
○ _____
○ _____
○ _____

✥ S U N • September 06, 2020

_____
_____
_____
_____
_____
_____
_____

○ _____
○ _____
○ _____
○ _____
○ _____
○ _____
○ _____

TO DO

_____
_____
_____
_____
_____

NOTE

○ _____
○ _____
○ _____
○ _____
○ _____
○ _____
○ _____

✦ M O N • September, 7 2020

_____

_____

_____

_____

_____

_____

LABOR DAY _____

○ _____
○ _____
○ _____
○ _____
○ _____
○ _____
○ _____

✦ T U E • September 08, 2020

_____

_____

_____

_____

_____

_____

_____

○ _____
○ _____
○ _____
○ _____
○ _____
○ _____
○ _____

✦ W E D • September 09, 2020

_____

_____

_____

_____

_____

_____

_____

○ _____
○ _____
○ _____
○ _____
○ _____
○ _____
○ _____

✦ T H U • September 10, 2020

_____

_____

_____

_____

_____

_____

_____

○ _____
○ _____
○ _____
○ _____
○ _____
○ _____
○ _____

✾ F R I • September 11, 2020

_____   ○ _____
_____   ○ _____
_____   ○ _____
_____   ○ _____
_____   ○ _____
_____   ○ _____
_____   ○ _____

✾ S A T • September 12, 2020

_____   ○ _____
_____   ○ _____
_____   ○ _____
_____   ○ _____
_____   ○ _____
_____   ○ _____
_____   ○ _____

✾ S U N • September 13, 2020

_____   ○ _____
_____   ○ _____
_____   ○ _____
_____   ○ _____
_____   ○ _____
_____   ○ _____
_____   ○ _____

TO DO   ## NOTE

_____   ○ _____
_____   ○ _____
_____   ○ _____
_____   ○ _____
_____   ○ _____
_____   ○ _____
_____   ○ _____

❖ M O N • September, 14 2020

_____   ○ _____
_____   ○ _____
_____   ○ _____
_____   ○ _____
_____   ○ _____
_____   ○ _____
_____   ○ _____

❖ T U E • September 15, 2020

_____   ○ _____
_____   ○ _____
_____   ○ _____
_____   ○ _____
_____   ○ _____
_____   ○ _____
_____   ○ _____

❖ W E D • September 16, 2020

_____   ○ _____
_____   ○ _____
_____   ○ _____
_____   ○ _____
_____   ○ _____
_____   ○ _____
_____   ○ _____

❖ T H U • September 17, 2020

_____   ○ _____
_____   ○ _____
_____   ○ _____
_____   ○ _____
_____   ○ _____
_____   ○ _____
_____   ○ _____

❈ F   R   I • September 18, 2020

_____   ◯ _____
_____   ◯ _____
_____   ◯ _____
_____   ◯ _____
_____   ◯ _____
_____   ◯ _____
_____   ◯ _____

❈ S   A   T • September 19, 2020

_____   ◯ _____
_____   ◯ _____
_____   ◯ _____
_____   ◯ _____
_____   ◯ _____
_____   ◯ _____
_____   ◯ _____

❈ S   U   N • September 20, 2020

_____   ◯ _____
_____   ◯ _____
_____   ◯ _____
_____   ◯ _____
_____   ◯ _____
_____   ◯ _____
_____   ◯ _____

TO DO   NOTE

_____   ◯ _____
_____   ◯ _____
_____   ◯ _____
_____   ◯ _____
_____   ◯ _____
_____   ◯ _____
_____   ◯ _____

✦ M O N • September, 21 2020

_____
_____   ○ _____
_____   ○ _____
_____   ○ _____
_____   ○ _____
_____   ○ _____
_____   ○ _____
_____   ○ _____

✦ T U E • September 22, 2020

_____
_____   ○ _____
_____   ○ _____
_____   ○ _____
_____   ○ _____
_____   ○ _____
_____   ○ _____
_____   ○ _____

✦ W E D • September 23, 2020

_____
_____   ○ _____
_____   ○ _____
_____   ○ _____
_____   ○ _____
_____   ○ _____
_____   ○ _____
_____   ○ _____

✦ T H U • September 24, 2020

_____
_____   ○ _____
_____   ○ _____
_____   ○ _____
_____   ○ _____
_____   ○ _____
_____   ○ _____
_____   ○ _____

❀ F R I • September 25, 2020

_____ ○ _____
_____ ○ _____
_____ ○ _____
_____ ○ _____
_____ ○ _____
_____ ○ _____
_____ ○ _____

❀ S A T • September 26, 2020

_____ ○ _____
_____ ○ _____
_____ ○ _____
_____ ○ _____
_____ ○ _____
_____ ○ _____
_____ ○ _____

❀ S U N • September 27, 2020

_____ ○ _____
_____ ○ _____
_____ ○ _____
_____ ○ _____
_____ ○ _____
_____ ○ _____
_____ ○ _____

TO DO   ## NOTE

_____ ○ _____
_____ ○ _____
_____ ○ _____
_____ ○ _____
_____ ○ _____
_____ ○ _____
_____ ○ _____

✦ M O N • September, 28 2020

_____   ◯ _____
_____   ◯ _____
_____   ◯ _____
_____   ◯ _____
_____   ◯ _____
_____   ◯ _____
_____   ◯ _____

✦ T U E • September 29, 2020

_____   ◯ _____
_____   ◯ _____
_____   ◯ _____
_____   ◯ _____
_____   ◯ _____
_____   ◯ _____
_____   ◯ _____

✦ W E D • September 30, 2020

_____   ◯ _____
_____   ◯ _____
_____   ◯ _____
_____   ◯ _____
_____   ◯ _____
_____   ◯ _____
_____   ◯ _____

✦ T H U • October 01, 2020

_____   ◯ _____
_____   ◯ _____
_____   ◯ _____
_____   ◯ _____
_____   ◯ _____
_____   ◯ _____
_____   ◯ _____

❖ F R I • October 02, 2020

_____   ○ _____
_____   ○ _____
_____   ○ _____
_____   ○ _____
_____   ○ _____
_____   ○ _____
_____   ○ _____

❖ S A T • October 03, 2020

_____   ○ _____
_____   ○ _____
_____   ○ _____
_____   ○ _____
_____   ○ _____
_____   ○ _____
_____   ○ _____

❖ S U N • October 04, 2020

_____   ○ _____
_____   ○ _____
_____   ○ _____
_____   ○ _____
_____   ○ _____
_____   ○ _____
_____   ○ _____

TO DO   ## NOTE

_____   ○ _____
_____   ○ _____
_____   ○ _____
_____   ○ _____
_____   ○ _____
_____   ○ _____
_____   ○ _____

❖ M O N • October, 5 2020

_____ ○ _____
_____ ○ _____
_____ ○ _____
_____ ○ _____
_____ ○ _____
_____ ○ _____
_____ ○ _____

❖ T U E • October 06, 2020

_____ ○ _____
_____ ○ _____
_____ ○ _____
_____ ○ _____
_____ ○ _____
_____ ○ _____
_____ ○ _____

❖ W E D • October 07, 2020

_____ ○ _____
_____ ○ _____
_____ ○ _____
_____ ○ _____
_____ ○ _____
_____ ○ _____
_____ ○ _____

❖ T H U • October 08, 2020

_____ ○ _____
_____ ○ _____
_____ ○ _____
_____ ○ _____
_____ ○ _____
_____ ○ _____
_____ ○ _____

FRI • October 09, 2020

_____   ○ _____
_____   ○ _____
_____   ○ _____
_____   ○ _____
_____   ○ _____
_____   ○ _____
_____   ○ _____

SAT • October 10, 2020

_____   ○ _____
_____   ○ _____
_____   ○ _____
_____   ○ _____
_____   ○ _____
_____   ○ _____
_____   ○ _____

SUN • October 11, 2020

_____   ○ _____
_____   ○ _____
_____   ○ _____
_____   ○ _____
_____   ○ _____
_____   ○ _____
_____   ○ _____

TO DO   ## NOTE

_____   ○ _____
_____   ○ _____
_____   ○ _____
_____   ○ _____
_____   ○ _____
_____   ○ _____
_____   ○ _____

❖ M O N • October, 12 2020

_____
_____
_____
_____
_____
_____
COLUMBUS DAY

○ _____
○ _____
○ _____
○ _____
○ _____
○ _____
○ _____

❖ T U E • October 13, 2020

_____
_____
_____
_____
_____
_____
_____

○ _____
○ _____
○ _____
○ _____
○ _____
○ _____
○ _____

❖ W E D • October 14, 2020

_____
_____
_____
_____
_____
_____
_____

○ _____
○ _____
○ _____
○ _____
○ _____
○ _____
○ _____

❖ T H U • October 15, 2020

_____
_____
_____
_____
_____

○ _____
○ _____
○ _____
○ _____
○ _____
○ _____
○ _____

❁ F R I • October 16, 2020

○
○
○
○
○
○
○

❁ S A T • October 17, 2020

○
○
○
○
○
○
○

❁ S U N • October 18, 2020

○
○
○
○
○
○
○

TO DO

NOTE

○
○
○
○
○
○
○

✦ M O N • October, 19 2020

_____
_____
_____
_____
_____
_____
_____

○ _____
○ _____
○ _____
○ _____
○ _____
○ _____
○ _____

✦ T U E • October 20, 2020

_____
_____
_____
_____
_____
_____
_____

○ _____
○ _____
○ _____
○ _____
○ _____
○ _____
○ _____

✦ W E D • October 21, 2020

_____
_____
_____
_____
_____
_____
_____

○ _____
○ _____
○ _____
○ _____
○ _____
○ _____
○ _____

✦ T H U • October 22, 2020

_____
_____
_____
_____
_____
_____
_____

○ _____
○ _____
○ _____
○ _____
○ _____
○ _____
○ _____

FRI • October 23, 2020

- _____
- _____
- _____
- _____
- _____
- _____
- _____

○ _____
○ _____
○ _____
○ _____
○ _____
○ _____
○ _____

SAT • October 24, 2020

- _____
- _____
- _____
- _____
- _____
- _____
- _____

○ _____
○ _____
○ _____
○ _____
○ _____
○ _____
○ _____

SUN • October 25, 2020

- _____
- _____
- _____
- _____
- _____
- _____
- _____

○ _____
○ _____
○ _____
○ _____
○ _____
○ _____
○ _____

TO DO

- _____
- _____
- _____
- _____
- _____

NOTE

○ _____
○ _____
○ _____
○ _____
○ _____
○ _____
○ _____

✤ M O N • October, 26 2020

_____   ○   _____
_____   ○   _____
_____   ○   _____
_____   ○   _____
_____   ○   _____
_____   ○   _____
_____   ○   _____

✤ T U E • October 27, 2020

_____   ○   _____
_____   ○   _____
_____   ○   _____
_____   ○   _____
_____   ○   _____
_____   ○   _____
_____   ○   _____

✤ W E D • October 28, 2020

_____   ○   _____
_____   ○   _____
_____   ○   _____
_____   ○   _____
_____   ○   _____
_____   ○   _____
_____   ○   _____

✤ T H U • October 29, 2020

_____   ○   _____
_____   ○   _____
_____   ○   _____
_____   ○   _____
_____   ○   _____
_____   ○   _____
_____   ○   _____

✦ F R I • October 30, 2020

_____
_____   ○ _____
_____   ○ _____
_____   ○ _____
_____   ○ _____
_____   ○ _____
_____   ○ _____
                                     ○ _____

✦ S A T • October 31, 2020

_____   ○ _____
_____   ○ _____
_____   ○ _____
_____   ○ _____
_____   ○ _____
_____   ○ _____
HALLOWEEN   ○ _____

✦ S U N • November 01, 2020

_____   ○ _____
_____   ○ _____
_____   ○ _____
_____   ○ _____
_____   ○ _____
_____   ○ _____
_____   ○ _____

TO DO   # NOTE

_____   ○ _____
_____   ○ _____
_____   ○ _____
_____   ○ _____
_____   ○ _____
_____   ○ _____
                                     ○ _____

❖ M O N • November, 2 2020

_____   ○ _____
_____   ○ _____
_____   ○ _____
_____   ○ _____
_____   ○ _____
_____   ○ _____
_____   ○ _____

❖ T U E • November 03, 2020

_____   ○ _____
_____   ○ _____
_____   ○ _____
_____   ○ _____
_____   ○ _____
_____   ○ _____
ELECTION DAY_____   ○ _____

❖ W E D • November 04, 2020

_____   ○ _____
_____   ○ _____
_____   ○ _____
_____   ○ _____
_____   ○ _____
_____   ○ _____
_____   ○ _____

❖ T H U • November 05, 2020

_____   ○ _____
_____   ○ _____
_____   ○ _____
_____   ○ _____
_____   ○ _____
_____   ○ _____
_____   ○ _____

� F R I • November 06, 2020

_____   ○ _____
_____   ○ _____
_____   ○ _____
_____   ○ _____
_____   ○ _____
_____   ○ _____
_____   ○ _____

✿ S A T • November 07, 2020

_____   ○ _____
_____   ○ _____
_____   ○ _____
_____   ○ _____
_____   ○ _____
_____   ○ _____
_____   ○ _____

✿ S U N • November 08, 2020

_____   ○ _____
_____   ○ _____
_____   ○ _____
_____   ○ _____
_____   ○ _____
_____   ○ _____
_____   ○ _____

TO DO   NOTE

_____   ○ _____
_____   ○ _____
_____   ○ _____
_____   ○ _____
_____   ○ _____
_____   ○ _____
                              ○ _____

MON • November, 9 2020

- _____
- _____
- _____
- _____
- _____
- _____
- _____

○ _____
○ _____
○ _____
○ _____
○ _____
○ _____
○ _____

TUE • November 10, 2020

- _____
- _____
- _____
- _____
- _____
- _____
- _____

○ _____
○ _____
○ _____
○ _____
○ _____
○ _____
○ _____

WED • November 11, 2020

- _____
- _____
- _____
- _____
- _____
- _____

VETERAN'S DAY

○ _____
○ _____
○ _____
○ _____
○ _____
○ _____
○ _____

THU • November 12, 2020

- _____
- _____
- _____
- _____
- _____

○ _____
○ _____
○ _____
○ _____
○ _____
○ _____
○ _____

✺ F R I • November 13, 2020

_____ ○ _____
_____ ○ _____
_____ ○ _____
_____ ○ _____
_____ ○ _____
_____ ○ _____
_____ ○ _____

✺ S A T • November 14, 2020

_____ ○ _____
_____ ○ _____
_____ ○ _____
_____ ○ _____
_____ ○ _____
_____ ○ _____
_____ ○ _____

✺ S U N • November 15, 2020

_____ ○ _____
_____ ○ _____
_____ ○ _____
_____ ○ _____
_____ ○ _____
_____ ○ _____
_____ ○ _____

TO DO   NOTE

_____ ○ _____
_____ ○ _____
_____ ○ _____
_____ ○ _____
_____ ○ _____
_____ ○ _____
_____ ○ _____

MON • November, 16 2020

_____   ○ _____
_____   ○ _____
_____   ○ _____
_____   ○ _____
_____   ○ _____
_____   ○ _____
_____   ○ _____

TUE • November 17, 2020

_____   ○ _____
_____   ○ _____
_____   ○ _____
_____   ○ _____
_____   ○ _____
_____   ○ _____
_____   ○ _____

WED • November 18, 2020

_____   ○ _____
_____   ○ _____
_____   ○ _____
_____   ○ _____
_____   ○ _____
_____   ○ _____
_____   ○ _____

THU • November 19, 2020

_____   ○ _____
_____   ○ _____
_____   ○ _____
_____   ○ _____
_____   ○ _____
_____   ○ _____
_____   ○ _____

✿ F   R   I • November 20, 2020

○
○
○
○
○
○
○

✿ S   A   T • November 21, 2020

○
○
○
○
○
○
○

✿ S   U   N • November 22, 2020

○
○
○
○
○
○
○

TO DO

NOTE

○
○
○
○
○
○
○

❋ M O N • November, 23 2020

_____ ◯ _____
_____ ◯ _____
_____ ◯ _____
_____ ◯ _____
_____ ◯ _____
_____ ◯ _____
_____ ◯ _____

❋ T U E • November 24, 2020

_____ ◯ _____
_____ ◯ _____
_____ ◯ _____
_____ ◯ _____
_____ ◯ _____
_____ ◯ _____
_____ ◯ _____

❋ W E D • November 25, 2020

_____ ◯ _____
_____ ◯ _____
_____ ◯ _____
_____ ◯ _____
_____ ◯ _____
_____ ◯ _____
_____ ◯ _____

❋ T H U • November 26, 2020

_____ ◯ _____
_____ ◯ _____
_____ ◯ _____
_____ ◯ _____
_____ ◯ _____
_____ ◯ _____
THANKSGIVING DAY   ◯ _____

F R I • November 27, 2020

BLACK FRIDAY

S A T • November 28, 2020

S U N • November 29, 2020

TO DO

NOTE

❀ M O N • November, 30 2020

_____   ○ _____
_____   ○ _____
_____   ○ _____
_____   ○ _____
_____   ○ _____
_____   ○ _____
_____   ○ _____

❀ T U E • December 01, 2020

_____   ○ _____
_____   ○ _____
_____   ○ _____
_____   ○ _____
_____   ○ _____
_____   ○ _____
_____   ○ _____

❀ W E D • December 02, 2020

_____   ○ _____
_____   ○ _____
_____   ○ _____
_____   ○ _____
_____   ○ _____
_____   ○ _____
_____   ○ _____

❀ T H U • December 03, 2020

_____   ○ _____
_____   ○ _____
_____   ○ _____
_____   ○ _____
_____   ○ _____
_____   ○ _____
_____   ○ _____

FRI • December 04, 2020

○
○
○
○
○
○
○

SAT • December 05, 2020

○
○
○
○
○
○
○

SUN • December 06, 2020

○
○
○
○
○
○
○

TO DO

NOTE

○
○
○
○
○
○
○

❖ M O N • December, 7 2020

_____
_____
_____   ○   _____
_____   ○   _____
_____   ○   _____
_____   ○   _____
_____   ○   _____
                              ○   _____
                              ○   _____
                              ○

❖ T U E • December 08, 2020

_____
_____   ○   _____
_____   ○   _____
_____   ○   _____
_____   ○   _____
_____   ○   _____
_____   ○   _____
_____   ○

❖ W E D • December 09, 2020

_____
_____   ○   _____
_____   ○   _____
_____   ○   _____
_____   ○   _____
_____   ○   _____
_____   ○   _____
_____   ○

❖ T H U • December 10, 2020

_____
_____   ○   _____
_____   ○   _____
_____   ○   _____
_____   ○   _____
_____   ○   _____
_____   ○   _____
                              ○

✦ F R I • December 11, 2020

- ◯
- ◯
- ◯
- ◯
- ◯
- ◯
- ◯

✦ S A T • December 12, 2020

- ◯
- ◯
- ◯
- ◯
- ◯
- ◯
- ◯

✦ S U N • December 13, 2020

- ◯
- ◯
- ◯
- ◯
- ◯
- ◯
- ◯

TO DO

NOTE

- ◯
- ◯
- ◯
- ◯
- ◯
- ◯
- ◯

✦ M O N • December, 14 2020

_____   ○
_____   ○ _____
_____   ○ _____
_____   ○ _____
_____   ○ _____
_____   ○ _____
_____   ○ _____
                            ○ _____

✦ T U E • December 15, 2020

_____   ○
_____   ○ _____
_____   ○ _____
_____   ○ _____
_____   ○ _____
_____   ○ _____
_____   ○ _____
                            ○ _____

✦ W E D • December 16, 2020

_____   ○
_____   ○ _____
_____   ○ _____
_____   ○ _____
_____   ○ _____
_____   ○ _____
_____   ○ _____
                            ○ _____

✦ T H U • December 17, 2020

_____   ○
_____   ○ _____
_____   ○ _____
_____   ○ _____
_____   ○ _____
_____   ○ _____
_____   ○ _____
                            ○ _____

✿ F R I • December 18, 2020

○
○
○
○
○
○
○

✿ S A T • December 19, 2020

○
○
○
○
○
○
○

✿ S U N • December 20, 2020

○
○
○
○
○
○
○

TO DO

NOTE

○
○
○
○
○
○
○

✦ M O N • December, 21 2020

_____   ○ _____
_____   ○ _____
_____   ○ _____
_____   ○ _____
_____   ○ _____
_____   ○ _____
_____   ○ _____

✦ T U E • December 22, 2020

_____   ○ _____
_____   ○ _____
_____   ○ _____
_____   ○ _____
_____   ○ _____
_____   ○ _____
_____   ○ _____

✦ W E D • December 23, 2020

_____   ○ _____
_____   ○ _____
_____   ○ _____
_____   ○ _____
_____   ○ _____
_____   ○ _____
_____   ○ _____

✦ T H U • December 24, 2020

_____   ○ _____
_____   ○ _____
_____   ○ _____
_____   ○ _____
_____   ○ _____
_____   ○ _____
CHRISTMAS EVE   ○ _____

✦ F R I • December 25, 2020

_____ ○ _____
_____ ○ _____
_____ ○ _____
_____ ○ _____
_____ ○ _____
_____ ○ _____
CHRISTMAS DAY _____ ○ _____

✦ S A T • December 26, 2020

_____ ○ _____
_____ ○ _____
_____ ○ _____
_____ ○ _____
_____ ○ _____
_____ ○ _____
_____ ○ _____

✦ S U N • December 27, 2020

_____ ○ _____
_____ ○ _____
_____ ○ _____
_____ ○ _____
_____ ○ _____
_____ ○ _____
_____ ○ _____

TO DO   ## NOTE

_____ ○ _____
_____ ○ _____
_____ ○ _____
_____ ○ _____
_____ ○ _____
_____ ○ _____
                          ○ _____

❀ M O N • December, 28 2020

_____ ○ _____
_____ ○ _____
_____ ○ _____
_____ ○ _____
_____ ○ _____
_____ ○ _____
_____ ○ _____

❀ T U E • December 29, 2020

_____ ○ _____
_____ ○ _____
_____ ○ _____
_____ ○ _____
_____ ○ _____
_____ ○ _____
_____ ○ _____

❀ W E D • December 30, 2020

_____ ○ _____
_____ ○ _____
_____ ○ _____
_____ ○ _____
_____ ○ _____
_____ ○ _____
_____ ○ _____

❀ T H U • December 31, 2020

_____ ○ _____
_____ ○ _____
_____ ○ _____
_____ ○ _____
_____ ○ _____
_____ ○ _____
NEW YEAR'S EVE _____ ○ _____

✿ F R I • January 01, 2021

_____
_____
_____
_____
_____
_____
NEW YEAR'S DAY

○ _____
○ _____
○ _____
○ _____
○ _____
○ _____
○ _____

✿ S A T • January 02, 2021

_____
_____
_____
_____
_____
_____
_____

○ _____
○ _____
○ _____
○ _____
○ _____
○ _____
○ _____

✿ S U N • January 03, 2021

_____
_____
_____
_____
_____
_____
_____

○ _____
○ _____
○ _____
○ _____
○ _____
○ _____
○ _____

TO DO

_____
_____
_____
_____
_____

NOTE

○ _____
○ _____
○ _____
○ _____
○ _____
○ _____
○ _____

NOTES

For more planners, journals and notebooks visit
www.nowpapergoods.com

Printed in Poland
by Amazon Fulfillment
Poland Sp. z o.o., Wrocław

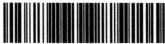